INTENTIONALLY

RED

A Definitive Guide for a Healthy Heart

Tamera McNeal, Ph.D

Table of Content

INTRODUCTION 5

CHAPTER ONE 11
  FEBRUARY NATIONAL HEART MONTH   11
    Symptoms of Heart Disease   16
    Symptoms of Heart Attack   16

CHAPTER TWO 21
  RISK AND CAUSES OF HEART DISEASES   21

CHAPTER THREE 31
  MANAGING HEART DISEASE   31

CHAPTER FOUR 39
  WAYS OF PREVENTING HEART DISEASE   39
    Top ten ways of preventing heart diseases 40

CHAPTER FIVE 49
  WHAT WE DO   49

CONCLUSION 65

REFERENCES....................................61

Introduction

When some people hear the words "heart disease", it sends chills down their spine. No one wants to be sick or plagued by a disease, because the majority of us love life and living. In February, we are going to put some of those fears to rest and raise awareness concerning one of the most vital aspects of human life. I'm dedicating this book, Intentionally Red, to people who have died of heart disease and those who are currently living with heart disease. I put this book together to share my personal experience with heart disease and to inspire you to take responsibility for your life, while staying informed.

So what you have here isn't just another book about heart disease but a much more detailed work that brings facts to you from my personal experience. I have a family history of hypertension, so the subject isn't new to me. After the birth of my last child on May 18, 2003, I woke up one morning to partial vision and limited mobility in my left arm and leg. I called the doctor who delivered my child, thinking the cause was related to my recent delivery. He advised me to return to the hospital, immediately. Once I arrived at the hospital and was examined, I was told I had suffered a stroke; it was one of the lowest points of my life. I was told that the stroke could have been caused by my elevated blood pressure. During the hospital stay, I was also diagnosed with heart disease. Oh, that was a whole lot of discouraging information coming all at once; I felt like a huge load of problems had been dropped on me, and I didn't know what steps to take going forward.

Sadly, after the health scare, I continued with my poor eating habits and didn't engage in any exercise. Guess what happened? My weight skyrocketed, which caused continuous elevated blood pressure readings, shortness of breath, chest pains and pressure on my knees. It wasn't until early 2013, after the death of my father, that I started taking my heart condition and health, seriously. I began to eat correctly while incorporating a good exercise regimen. Guess what happened? I ended up losing over 90lbs.

Although heart disease is something I will probably live with forever, my hypertension is under control, and the irregular heartbeats, shortness of breath and chest pains have all diminished.

I am in the best shape I have ever been, and my entire life has taken a turn for the best. I am so confident about my future because I decided to make some changes, and I want to share how you can make necessary health changes, too. For Heart Awareness month, I want you to prepare to learn more about your heart, because a healthy heart is vital to living a great life. Once you have read this book, your pool of knowledge will increase, and you will be in a better position to take decisive steps toward heart health. So many people admit to having limited information in regard to heart health awareness, thus, I was prompted to make information gathered through my research, available. All right, let's begin now with February, National Heart Disease month, and what heart disease is all about.

.

Chapter One

FEBRUARY: NATIONAL HEART MONTH

America designated February as Heart Month; it presents an opportunity to raise awareness of possible steps people can take to protect themselves from experiencing the leading cause of death in men and women in the United States (Heart Disease Facts, 2017). The situation worsens by the day, as it is reported that one in every four deaths is caused by heart disease (Heart Disease Facts, 2017). So what exactly is heart disease? Heart disease refers to a series of issues that affect the heart, such as a congenital heart defect or coronary artery disease.

Just like other muscles in the body, the heart needs the right supply of blood to aid oxygen flow so the muscles can pump blood to the essential parts of the body. The blood is pumped through the coronary arteries; these arteries originate from the base of the aorta, which is the main blood vessel that carries blood from the heart to its surface. Now, if any of the coronary arteries are narrowed, it makes it difficult for blood to get to the heart; the narrower the passage, the more difficult blood passage becomes, leading to cases of chest pain, shortness of breath and atherosclerotic heart disease.

If the arteries become blocked, it affects the supply of blood to the heart, causing a piece of the heart muscle to die; this is when heart attacks take place. At this point, you might begin to wonder how the blockage happens; what leads to such malfunctions and other questions may be on your mind as well. We will handle all of these and more as we proceed in the book. I just wanted to give you a glimpse into what happens in the heart, to help form a picture in your mind.

Sometimes, what is known as heart disease is called cardiovascular disease because it entails the blockage of blood vessels, preventing the proper circulation of blood and leading to a heart attack. However, you can avoid heart disease just by making healthy choices and living a life that reflects the right lifestyle choices. So many people still do not know that the choices they make in life affect the stress they put their heart through; as such, they end up doing things that have a direct, negative effect on their heart.

Heart disease is a lifelong condition that cannot be cured with medication; however, a successful heart bypass surgery will make it is possible for a person to get the proper flow of blood and oxygen to the heart. Nevertheless, the arteries in the center will be damaged for life, thus increasing the chance of having a heart attack. A lot of women die from heart attacks or complications from heart disease, so it is imperative for women to observe, take action, and control the disease.

Because many people only have the basic information about heart disease, dedicating an entire month to raising awareness and sharing thoughts in regard to this condition is one way we all can reach out to those who aren't aware. So in February, you can reach out to others with this book and try to help them to understand that whatever process they allow their heart to pass through will ultimately affect its health. Having gained an understanding into what heart disease is about and the process it takes, I want you to understand the symptoms that often give signs that a person has heart disease and the symptoms of a heart attack, as well. Remember that this book is a complete guide to help you know all about heart disease, so let's look at the possible symptoms; shall we?

SYMPTOMS OF HEART DISEASE

- A faster heartbeat
- Nausea
- Shortness of breath
- Sweating
- Palpations

SYMPTOMS OF HEART ATTACK

- Vomiting
- Dizziness
- Extreme weakness
- Rapid or irregular heartbeats
- Shortness of breath
- Sweating
- Discomfort (feeling of heartburn)

However, you should know that some people experience heart attacks without actually showing these symptoms. In such cases, it is called a silent myocardial ischaemia (SMI), which is the common cause of mortality in people with diabetes (Royal Alexandra

Hospital, 1999). As you become familiar with your body, you will receive signs that will help you know what to do and when to do it. For heart disease to be diagnosed, a health care professional will have to look into the patient's health history and understand the kinds of symptoms that have manifested.

Sometimes the symptoms may be mistaken for something else, so it is essential that if you feel any of the symptoms above, be clear in your description, so your physician knows exactly what's wrong and can offer solutions, accordingly. The factors surrounding the signs will also give a better clue to what may be wrong, so ask yourself questions like: Are these symptoms caused by activity or inactivity? Do you experience relief when you rest? Do the signs make it difficult to sleep? These questions will also help in the identification of risk factors (we will shed more light on this in subsequent chapters).

Understanding your body is key to getting the help you need when faced with heart disease; you need to be observant while examining your lifestyle choices, as well. Some people take a nonchalant approach to their personal health; they are not informed with regard to what happens in their body and so it becomes difficult for them to trace the emergence of symptoms. As we proceed to other chapters, I urge to take the time to look closely at your health and do a little research on your family's health history so you will be able to trace your own history. The next chapter looks at the

risks and causes of heart disease. With
your knowledge of what heart disease is
all about, you will become familiar with
the risk factors and activities or non-
activities that lead to heart disease.

.

Chapter Two

RISK AND CAUSES OF HEART DISEASES

To understand the solutions to heart diseases, we have to gain insight into what leads to the disease in the first place. This chapter examines the most likely risks for and causes of heart diseases, answers the questions "why" and "how", and gives direction to the quest to lower the cases of heart disease to the barest minimum. Some of the causes and risks will come as a surprise to you because you probably never thought these things could contribute. However, others will not be surprising because you probably already knew that they were risk factors. Some of these factors can be controlled while others cannot be controlled, so read on as I share the top ten causes of heart disease.

1. High Blood Cholesterol

Too much cholesterol in your blood affects the walls of your arteries, causing a process called atherosclerosis, which is a form of heart disease. The arteries become very narrow and this slows down the flow of blood being carried to the heart. At this point, you will suffer from chest pain and if the supply of blood is completely blocked out, it will lead to a heart attack.

2. The Age of the Individual

The risk of developing heart disease increases as you grow older. Most cardiovascular conditions occur in people who are over the age of 65. The most straightforward explanation for this is the fact that as we grow older, our blood vessels become more easily damaged, and the muscles around the heart also thicken, which it makes very difficult for the heart to pump blood as it should.

3. Gender

Initially, more men are at risk of getting heart disease than women, although it evens out as we grow older. Estrogen in women helps provide a preventive measure for them before they reach menopause; however, women face greater risk once they reach menopause and the level of estrogen production reduces. As such, by age 65 both men and women are exposed to high risk of getting heart disease.

4. Obesity

When a person is obese it increases the chances of developing heart disease. As a person carries extra weight around, it adds to the burden of pumping blood throughout the body. Obesity also causes high blood pressure, so it is essential that everyone watches their weight. Once you feel slightly obese, you should take action towards toning it down because the more overweight you are, the more you put yourself at risk.

5. Diabetes

Diabetes causes a lot of other diseases, and it comes in two forms; type

1, which is developed in those who are genetically predisposed to it and type 2 for those who develop it due to lack of proper exercise, diet and other factors. Diabetes can lead to plaque in the arteries, thus making it difficult for blood to flow through the body.

6. Family History

Some people are genetically linked to certain diseases. If you have a father who suffered from heart disease before the age of 65, then you stand a higher chance of getting it, as well. But it is worth noting that your lifestyle choices also play a crucial role; individuals who smoke, drink alcohol beverages or indulge in other unhealthy activities will also be at higher risk, with the family history still a significant factor.

7.   Deficiency in proper diet

You are a reflection of what you eat. If a person is genetically predisposed to getting heart disease and you are not, it doesn't mean you should be relaxed about your diet. Watch what you eat because goes in your body controls what happens in your body. Avoid foods that are high in saturated fat and salty foods. Eat a balanced diet, eat plenty of fruits and vegetables, and if you must drink alcohol beverages, it should be done responsibly.

8. Poor Hygiene

Hygiene is so important in this discourse. Wash your hands regularly, brush your teeth properly, and do whatever you must do to ensure that you are always clean because the outside also controls the narrative on the inside. It has been said that periodontal disease can increase your risk to heart disease, because if bacteria from periodontal disease spreads to your heart, it can cause inflammation. Check your environment and the activities you indulge in regularly. The kinds of precautions you take regarding hygiene play an important role in determining if you will be exposed to heart disease.

9. Lifestyle Choices

If you decide to drink alcoholic beverages and smoke often, then you are putting yourself at a higher risk of developing heart disease. Nicotine found in cigarettes constricts the blood vessels and the carbon monoxide can over time affect the blood vessels, thus putting smokers at higher risk of developing heart disease.

10. Hypertension

This is also known as high blood pressure. If you consistently have high blood pressure then your arteries will thicken, thus shrinking the blood vessels and making it extremely difficult for the heart to pump blood throughout the body. Some people aren't aware that they have high blood pressure, increasing the risk of heart attacks people have without having symptoms.

The causes mentioned may or may not be new to you. Regardless of how new the information is, you must take decisive steps to ensure that these factors are examined correctly. The key to getting rid of any problem is to understand its nature then work toward eliminating it. My vision for this book is that by the time you are done reading, you will be empowered not only to know more about the heart but also to be able to reach out to others and educate them on what they need to do to live a much healthier life. The next chapter focuses on how to best manage heart disease, should it happen; read on.

Chapter Three

MANAGING HEART DISEASE

Should you develop heart disease, you will need to know how to best handle it. This chapter will help you identify the most effective steps you can take to manage heart disease so that you will remain in favorable health condition for a longer time. Despite the fact that there is no specific cure for heart disease, you can take little steps daily toward helping yourself manage the situation. You will need help from others, and you will have to get rid of certain habits that aren't consistent with what you desire for yourself but through it all, have faith that you will come out better and stronger.

I still live with my heart condition, but I can tell you that with the steps I'm about to share with you, I live a happier life, filled with purpose and direction. You don't have to drown in depression, and you don't have to start feeling sorry for yourself; there is so much more life left in you. So let's highlight some of the essential ways through which heart disease can be managed; shall we?

• **Make Changes**

Everything about managing heart disease begins and ends with your lifestyle, so if you are saying you want to maintain your health correctly, then you have to start by making some very swift changes in that direction. If you smoke, then it's time to quit; if you're not eating properly, then you need to start; if you weren't exercising enough, then it's time to visit the gym or local park. Your life, at this point, should be all about change and how the change is going to help you feel better every day.

• **Set Realistic Goals**

At this point, you've got to have health goals. What do you want to see happen in your life, and what do you want to achieve now that you have this disease? These questions should drive you into setting goals and writing those goals out; make it understandable, as this will help you do something about them. I set a goal for myself that entailed me getting enough sleep, as recommended by my doctor. I did my best to ensure that the goal was achieved, and today I sleep better because I know that proper rest is essential to good health.

• **Track your Goals**

After setting goals, the next thing to do is to track your goals, making sure you are doing what you are supposed to do. The best way to track your goals is to set a deadline, so it shouldn't just be about you writing out a goal; it should be about you making efforts to fulfill the goal. You are somewhat responsible for what happens to you so try your best by following through with everything related to your goals. I was able to track my goals by getting a journal where I wrote down the progress I made for the week and the month; gradually, it became a huge part of my life, and now implement those things I set as goals without actually checking the journal—how sweet!

• Prepare for setbacks

This is inevitable! Your body is probably already used to a particular routine, as such, so when you introduce something new, it will rebel and fight it off at first, but here's a secret: if you persist enough, you will overpower your body and win. So be prepared for setbacks at some point but don't be perturbed about it. If you fall, merely pick yourself up, again, and you will be just fine. However, once you are prepared for them, it gets easier and it helps if you know exactly what to expect.

• Give yourself time

You are probably feeling so down and sad about this disease, but you have to give yourself time. You have to be patient with yourself and allow yourself to make mistakes. The heart disease will change your thought process, and you will find yourself with a feeling of sadness, but I can assure you from experience that everything will be just fine once you give yourself time to believe again and build confidence in knowing you have everything within you to win.

• Maintain good social connections

Now more than ever, you need the help of your nearest and dearest. You need family and friends around you who will support you and help you go through this process. This isn't the time to run away from your friends and family; this is the time to accept shoulders to lean on while looking forward to a better life. Your social connections should be deepened at this point, and you have to trust the people around you to cheer you up when you feel unhappy.

• Be Optimistic

Of all the points here, this one trumps all. You need to be optimistic about life and remain positive, because if you cannot do anything about it, then you owe it to yourself to be happy. Be positive, trust life and be patient having faith that your healthy heart is being restored.

It has been a great chapter thus far, and I believe you have gleaned a lot, but more importantly, I want you to know that these steps will always be practical whenever you put them to good use. Look beyond what you see and feel right now and have faith that you can live a great life, regardless of this disease. The next chapter introduces the concept of prevention, which is one of the most critical message embedded in this book; you've got to know what to do to prevent the occurrence of heart disease.

Chapter Four

WAYS OF PREVENTING HEART DISEASE

Prevention is much better than frantically searching for a cure. If you can prevent the disease from happening, you will save more time and resources than if you have to seek a cure. So in this chapter, we will learn about how you can possibly prevent heart disease. Hopefully you will never have to go through what I went through; rather, you can start today by taking steps in the right direction and building a life that is healthy. There are a lot of things you can do to prevent heart disease; just stay tuned to this chapter, and you will learn the best ways to live.

TOP TEN WAYS OF PREVENTING HEART DISEASE

1. Check your Cholesterol level

Your level of cholesterol is affected by the types of food you eat, your weight, level of activity, age, family history and even certain diseases. Don't eat meals that are high in full fat, such as packaged foods, chips, cookies, etc. If you want to prevent heart disease, you've got to know how to assess what you eat at all times, because this is a major factor in determining if a person will develop heart disease or not.

2. Make sure your blood pressure is okay

This is also very important; as healthy blood pressure helps you from developing heart disease. High blood pressure is dangerous to your heart because it makes the heart work too hard for longer, thus damaging the arteries and making it impossible for blood to flow easily. Regular blood pressure checks are very good for your health, and you will be grateful for such checks because they help you keep tabs on your heart.

3. Don't smoke

You've probably heard this before; smoking isn't healthy, nor is it good for your heart. Avoid smoking, and you will not have to worry about heart disease if every other risk factor has been eliminated. If you smoke, then you should stop quickly because the longer you continue, the worse things will get for your heart.

4. Know what you are exposed to

What are some of the risks you are currently exposed to? Is it an environmental risk? Are they health hazards? You've got to know exactly what you are exposed to and cut these things out of your life for good. You cannot afford to stop checking on yourself because it is the only way you will be able to know what to let go of and what to incorporate. If you can recognize what you are exposed to, then you will know how to prevent it from affecting your heart.

5. Be health conscious

Being health conscious isn't just about getting regular checkups and knowing if all is well with your health. Being health conscious means you are willing to take the right steps for your health at all times, and you are willing to put your health first! Now, it may not be convenient for you, but this isn't about fun or convenience; this is about doing what is right.

6. Reduce stress

If you are stressed out, then chances are you are overworking your arteries as well. Try not to allow stress in! Maintain a productive life but don't allow yourself to get to the level of being so stressed out that you don't take time out to get your rest. The best and easiest way of preventing heart disease is by staying stress-free and just keeping a very positive outlook on life.

7. Be knowledgeable

By reading this book, you are gaining knowledge, but don't stop here. The month of February is about heart disease awareness, so there will be a lot of material out there for you, and you will get to read lots and lots of material on how to be mindful of heart disease. Take advantage of this and update your knowledge; when you are knowledgeable, it will lower your chances of being a victim.

8. Be careful in your use of non-prescription drugs

Some people tend to abuse drugs with hopes of curing their illness.

Some seek non-prescription drugs to enhance the performance of the heart, but this shouldn't be the case. If you get recommendations from a specialist, then it's fine, but please don't start using or abusing non-prescription drugs because you want to get your heart to beat at a certain rate or to with hopes of curing your heart disease.

9. Exercise is key

The heart needs to stay fit as well; it needs to get used to being stretched out, so exercise is key at this point. Ensure that you exercise enough and you devote enough time to put your body through the process, because people who do not exercise stand a higher risk of getting heart disease. It might be a walk down the street, using the stairs instead of the elevator—just do the simple things that put the body in motion.

10.   WATCH YOUR CALORIES

I cannot emphasize this enough! We've talked about cholesterol and how food is important in regard to your heart health; you should watch your calories, as well. Remember that your heart functions off what you feed it and the activities you indulge in, so whatever you eat and whatever you do must be done to protect your heart at all costs. So watch your calories, and exercise; whatever you do, please just always put your heart first!

I am so excited to bring this chapter to a close because I know that we have successfully considered just about every aspect of heart disease, ranging from the causes, the effects, ways to manage it and even the solutions. Now you know what to do, what to eat, drink and how to live because you have received a complete guide to everything that pertains to heart disease. In the next chapter, I will be sharing some of the work we do and how we are contributing to making the situation better.

Tamera McNeal, PhD

Chapter Five

WHAT WE DO

The CIARA Foundation is helping individuals

The CIARA (Critical Illness Awareness Research and Aid) Foundation is helping individuals fight heart disease, as well as other critical illnesses, and we need your help to make this work. When you visit www.CiaraFoundation.com, you will find information on how you can help other people who go through this disease. It is a platform through which you can give and make a difference so that wherever you are, you can put a smile on someone's face and lighten the burden that comes with battling heart disease, as well as other illnesses

Heart disease is the nation's number one killer disease, and stroke is the nation's number four killer disease. Such statistics call for action that will help the people affected get better health care as well as increased knowledge of what can be done to reduce the number of people who die from this disease, yearly. Your donation will help our life-saving efforts and also make it possible for anyone who has experienced these issues to reach out to others as well. Our organization assists with medication, medical transportation, medical equipment, medical scholarships, and more.

There are many ways you can give to the CIARA Foundation, and in this chapter, we will explore some of these ideas and provide a myriad of options, all tailored to suit your preferences. You will be amazed at the options available to you and the means through which your money can be channeled appropriately to help those in need; read more below.

1. Honoring a loved one

You can donate via this medium by creating a personal fundraising page. After creating your page, you have to tell your friends and loved ones about the page. Inform them that you are collecting funds on behalf of the CIARA Foundation for Heart Disease Awareness. As they donate, we can generate money which helps us reach out to persons who suffer from heart disease.

2. Help save lives monthly

You can be a monthly contributor by dedicating a particular sum of money to the cause. You can join in the fight to build a world that is heart disease-free through a monthly gift and support year-round to save lives.

3. Creating an event

FUNraise for heart disease and stroke and you will watch yourself having fun while making a massive difference in the lives of others. Create your fundraising page and start a holiday gift card asking your friends to forgo the usual gifts and support your page instead.

4. Other ways to give

There are different ways to give that are just right for you. There's the fun way that includes organizing a car wash event, a marathon or something unique that works for you. There is also the dear neighbor campaign, and vehicle donation, as well as the Heritage brick wall; discover ways through which you can add value to the campaign.

5. Schools

Kids can become empowered to give as well as become aware of the ways to keep fit for the future through Jump Rope for Heart and Hoops for Heart Help. The children can ask family and friends for donations while learning firsthand the importance of being generous to a worthy cause.

6. Sponsorship Opportunities

Your dollars can begin to work for you through research. With research needing lots of funds, it is our best option when it comes to seeking solutions for the future. Our goal is to be at the forefront of eradicating this menacing disease.

We can do nothing without you

Without you, we can do nothing. You are a very vital part of what we do, and this chapter is dedicated to you. We want you to know that we are always grateful to receive whatever you send and use it for the good of humanity and the preservation of our generation.

I decided to dedicate a chapter to this, so you'll become more aware of the work we are doing and how we are connecting lives and making things happen on a larger scale. I implore you to visit the site and make an effort to give through any of the categories that

appeal to you, as you are already familiar
with them from this chapter. .

Conclusion

bring this book to a fantastic end with JOY in my heart. It has been the most fantastic experience, and I cannot wait for you to start putting all you have learned to good use. We started this discourse by giving insight into what heart disease is all about and what you need to know about this condition that is taking many lives.

We also considered the rate at which people die from this disease, thus necessitating a heart month, which happens to be February. This book will serve as a guide because it is a detailed work on all things regarding heart disease.

We also talked about ways through which the disease manifests itself, which refers to the symptoms, as well as the best ways to manage such conditions if they occur. The preventive measures weren't left out, and we considered what we have done thus far as an organization. You can give toward supporting this cause and know that your funds will help fund research, education, advocating for better health, improve patient care and reach the populations at risk. I believe that everything you have learned here has prepared you not just to protect yourself, but to help others who might be in dire need.

So what will you do with everything

you have learned thus far? Are you going to keep the information to yourself until you see someone who needs it, or are you going to take action? You can reach out to those who are not informed and help them make healthier choices, because once a person develops heart disease, it will be difficult for him/her to go back to a normal life. I feel so blessed that I have an opportunity to share my journey with you, and I hope you will help put a smile on someone's face by contributing to a worthy cause.

I hope you will live a very healthy life that is backed by great habits and activities because of what you have read today. If you are already battling with heart disease, then you can manage it, and if you don't have it, you now know ways you can avoid it. Further, in

February, you can join in the awareness programs by purchasing products and material from the CIARA Foundation, making a donation to the organization and sharing our content with all. There is nothing you cannot achieve when you have knowledge. So get up and strategize on ways you can help share this message, as the world will be a better place when people help people.

References

Alexandra Hospital, P. U., R. (1999, July 13). National Library of Medicine - National Institutes of Health. Retrieved from https://www.nlm.nih.gov/

W. (n.d.). Retrieved February 05, 2018, from https://www.coursehero.com/file/p44cp3d9/a-Coronary-arteries-originate-from-the-base-of-the-aorta-just-above-the-aorc/

Writer, R. S. (2017, December 20). Retrieved February 05, 2018, from https://goodthingstoknow.co/heart-disease-symptoms-risk-causes/

(n.d.). Retrieved February 05, 2018, from
https://my.clevelandclinic.org/
health/diseases/17519-stroke

(n.d.). Retrieved February 05, 2018, from
https://wexnermedical.osu.edu/
heart-vascular/preventing-heart-
disease

(n.d.). Retrieved February 05, 2018,
from https://www.healthypeople.
gov/2020/topics-objectives/topic/
heart-disease-and-stroke

(n.d.). Retrieved February 05, 2018, from
https://www.nhlbi.nih.gov/health-
topics/heart-disease-women

(n.d.). Retrieved February 05, 2018,
from https://www.webmd.com/
cholesterol-management/tc/high-
cholesterol-overview

NOTES

NOTES